CANCER PREVENTION DIET COOKBOOK

Nourishing Recipes and Expert Guidance for Harnessing the Power of Nutrition in Your Fight Against Cancer

Dr. Holmgren Alfred

The "Cancer Prevention Diet Cookbook: With Expert Guidance" is not just another culinary guide; it's a powerful tool designed to empower individuals in their journey towards a healthier, cancer-free lifestyle.

As we navigate the complexities of modern living, understanding the intersection between diet and cancer prevention becomes increasingly vital. This book serves as a beacon of knowledge, shedding light on the pivotal role nutrition plays in safeguarding our well-being.

Within these pages, you'll embark on a comprehensive exploration of the intricate relationship between diet and cancer prevention. From deciphering the fundamentals of cancer prevention strategies to uncovering the key nutrients essential for fortifying our bodies against this formidable adversary, each chapter is meticulously crafted to arm readers with invaluable insights.

Delving deeper, you'll discover practical tips and strategies for transforming your kitchen into a formidable fortress against cancer. Learn how to stock your pantry with wholesome ingredients, master essential kitchen tools, and navigate the aisles with confidence, selecting foods renowned for their cancer-fighting properties.

But the true essence of this book lies in its culinary offerings—a tantalizing array of recipes meticulously curated to tantalize the taste buds while nurturing the body.

From nutrient-packed breakfast smoothies to wholesome dinners bursting with flavor, each dish is thoughtfully designed to harness the power of nature's bounty in the fight against cancer.

Moreover, this book transcends mere recipes; it's a roadmap to long-term success. Dive into meal planning strategies, discover the art of balanced meal plans, and glean insights on navigating social occasions without compromising your health goals. With expert guidance and unwavering support, you'll find yourself equipped not just with recipes, but with the knowledge and motivation needed to embark on a transformative journey towards optimal health.

In essence, the "Cancer Prevention Diet Cookbook: With Expert Guidance" is more than just a culinary compendium—it's a beacon of hope, a testament to the transformative power of nutrition, and a steadfast companion in your quest for a vibrant, cancer-free life.

Copyright © Holmgren Alfred 2024.

All rights reserved.

This book is fictitious. Authors create names, people, places, and events.

Any resemblance to real events, places, or people—living or dead—is coincidental.

DISCLAIMER

The information provided in this book, titled "Cancer Prevention: With Expert Guidance," is intended for informational purposes only and should not be construed as medical advice. The content presented herein is based on research, expert opinions, and general knowledge related to cancer prevention. However, it is not a substitute for professional medical advice, diagnosis, or treatment.

The author of this book makes no endorsements, representations, or warranties of any kind regarding the accuracy, completeness, or suitability of the information provided. Any references to individuals, products, websites, organizations, or other names are for informational purposes only and do not imply endorsement.

The inclusion of such references does not constitute an endorsement or recommendation by the author.

Readers are encouraged to consult with qualified healthcare professionals regarding any questions or concerns they may have about their health or any medical conditions. The author and publisher disclaim any liability for any loss, injury, or damage incurred as a consequence of the use or application of the information presented in this book.

By reading this book, you acknowledge and agree to the terms of this disclaimer.

INTRODUCTION

The introduction sets the stage for the reader, providing an overview of what they can expect from the book. It typically includes a brief explanation of the purpose of the book, its target audience, and what the reader stands to gain from it. In the case of the "Cancer Prevention Diet Cookbook," the introduction may begin by addressing the prevalence of cancer in modern society and the growing interest in preventive measures, including dietary interventions.

It may also touch upon the importance of nutrition in overall health and well-being, particularly in the context of cancer prevention.

Furthermore, the introduction could outline the structure of the cookbook, highlighting its focus on providing nourishing recipes and expert guidance for utilizing the power of nutrition in the fight against cancer.

 By offering a glimpse into the content and objectives of the book, the introduction serves to engage the reader and motivate them to explore further.

Understanding Cancer And Diet:

This section delves into the complex relationship between cancer and diet, aiming to educate the reader on the role that nutrition plays in both the development and prevention of cancer. It may begin by providing a brief overview of cancer as a disease, including its various forms, risk factors, and underlying mechanisms.

From there, the focus shifts to the influence of diet on cancer risk, highlighting how certain dietary patterns and food choices can either promote or inhibit the development of cancerous cells.

For instance, the discussion may touch upon the importance of consuming a balanced diet rich in fruits, vegetables, whole grains, and lean proteins, while minimizing intake of processed foods, red meat, and sugary beverages.

Additionally, this section may explore specific nutrients and bioactive compounds found in foods that have been linked to cancer prevention, such as antioxidants, phytochemicals, and omega-3 fatty acids. By providing evidence-based insights into the relationship between cancer and diet, this section empowers readers to make informed choices about their eating habits to reduce their risk of developing cancer.

Importance Of Nutrition In Cancer Prevention:

Building upon the foundation laid in the previous section, the importance of nutrition in cancer prevention is further emphasized and elucidated. Here, the focus is on elucidating the mechanisms through which dietary factors can influence various stages of cancer development, from initiation to progression and metastasis. This may involve discussing the impact of specific nutrients on key biological processes such as inflammation, oxidative stress, DNA damage, and hormonal regulation, all of which play critical roles in carcinogenesis. Moreover, this section may address the concept of "nutritional oncology," which explores the use of dietary interventions as adjunctive therapies for cancer treatment and management. By highlighting the potential of nutrition to modulate the tumor microenvironment, enhance immune function, and improve treatment outcomes, readers are encouraged to view dietary modifications as a proactive strategy for reducing cancer risk and optimizing health. Additionally, the importance of adopting a holistic approach to nutrition, encompassing not only food choices but also lifestyle factors such as physical activity, stress management, and sleep hygiene, may be emphasized to underscore the multifaceted nature of cancer prevention.

How This Cookbook Can Help:

In this final section, the focus shifts to the practical application of the preceding information, outlining how the cookbook serves as a valuable resource for individuals seeking to implement dietary changes in support of cancer prevention.

Here, the unique features and benefits of the cookbook are highlighted, such as its collection of nourishing recipes specifically designed to incorporate cancer-fighting ingredients and culinary techniques. Readers are introduced to the diverse range of dishes included in the cookbook, which may encompass everything from antioxidant-rich smoothies and vibrant salads to hearty soups and flavorful entrees. Additionally, the expertise of the contributing authors or consultants, whether they be nutritionists, dietitians, oncologists, or chefs, is showcased to lend credibility to the content and recommendations provided. Moreover, the practical tips, meal planning guides, and educational resources interspersed throughout the cookbook are underscored as valuable tools for empowering readers to make sustainable dietary changes. By offering a comprehensive yet accessible approach to cancer prevention through nutrition, the cookbook aims to inspire and support readers on their journey toward optimal health and well-being.

CHAPTER 1
THE BASICS OF CANCER PREVENTION

Cancer prevention is a multifaceted approach aimed at reducing the risk of developing cancer through various strategies, including lifestyle modifications, dietary changes, screening, and vaccination. Understanding the basics of cancer prevention involves recognizing the factors that contribute to the development of cancer, such as genetics, environmental exposures, and lifestyle choices.

By targeting these factors, individuals can adopt proactive measures to lower their risk of cancer and promote overall health and well-being.

Overview Of Cancer Prevention Strategies:

Cancer prevention strategies encompass a range of interventions designed to mitigate the risk factors associated with cancer development. These strategies often involve lifestyle modifications, including smoking cessation, maintaining a healthy weight, regular physical activity, limiting alcohol consumption, and protecting against exposure to harmful substances such as UV radiation and environmental carcinogens. Additionally, screening tests and vaccination programs play a crucial role in the early detection and prevention of certain cancers, allowing for prompt treatment and improved outcomes. By implementing comprehensive prevention strategies, individuals can significantly reduce their risk of developing cancer and enhance their quality of life.

Role Of Diet In Cancer Prevention:

Diet plays a pivotal role in cancer prevention, as research indicates that certain dietary patterns and food choices can influence the development and progression of various types of cancer.

A diet rich in fruits, vegetables, whole grains, and lean proteins provides essential nutrients, antioxidants, and phytochemicals that help protect against cancer by promoting cellular health, supporting immune function, and reducing inflammation. Conversely, diets high in processed foods, red and processed meats, saturated fats, and sugary beverages have been linked to an increased risk of cancer. By adopting a balanced and nutrient-dense diet, individuals can optimize their body's defenses against cancer and promote overall well-being.

Key Nutrients For Cancer Prevention:

Several key nutrients have been identified for their potential role in cancer prevention, including vitamins, minerals, antioxidants, and phytochemicals.

Vitamin D, for example, plays a critical role in regulating cell growth and immune function, and adequate levels have been associated with a reduced risk of certain cancers, such as colorectal and breast cancer.

Similarly, antioxidants like vitamin C, vitamin E, and selenium help neutralize harmful free radicals, which can damage cells and contribute to cancer development. Phytochemicals found in plant-based foods, such as flavonoids, carotenoids, and polyphenols, possess anti-inflammatory and antioxidant properties that can inhibit cancer growth and metastasis.

Additionally, dietary fiber, omega-3 fatty acids, and probiotics have been shown to exert protective effects against cancer by promoting digestive health and modulating immune function. By incorporating a diverse range of nutrient-rich foods into their diet, individuals can optimize their intake of these essential nutrients and reduce their risk of cancer.

CHAPTER 2
BUILDING A CANCER-FIGHTING KITCHEN

Creating a cancer-fighting kitchen involves a multifaceted approach that integrates both nutritional knowledge and practical cooking techniques. The concept encompasses not only the selection of specific foods known for their cancer-preventive properties but also the organization of the kitchen space and the adoption of cooking practices that maximize the retention of nutrients.

A key aspect of this concept involves understanding the role of various food components, such as antioxidants, phytochemicals, fiber, and healthy fats, in protecting cells from damage and promoting overall health. Moreover, a cancer-fighting kitchen emphasizes the incorporation of a diverse range of fruits, vegetables, whole grains, legumes, nuts, and seeds into daily meals, as these foods are rich sources of vitamins, minerals, and bioactive compounds that support the body's natural defense mechanisms against cancer development. Additionally, attention is paid to minimizing the consumption of processed and refined foods, which often contain additives and preservatives that may have adverse effects on health.

By adopting a cancer-fighting kitchen approach, individuals can not only enhance their nutritional intake but also cultivate sustainable dietary habits that contribute to long-term well-being and disease prevention.

Stocking Your Pantry For Cancer Prevention:

Stocking a pantry for cancer prevention involves strategically selecting and storing a variety of nutrient-dense foods that support overall health and reduce the risk of cancer development. This process begins with the identification of foods that are rich in antioxidants, phytochemicals, vitamins, and minerals, which play crucial roles in neutralizing harmful free radicals, regulating cell growth, and supporting immune function. Examples of such foods include colorful fruits and vegetables like berries, leafy greens, cruciferous vegetables, and citrus fruits, as well as whole grains, legumes, nuts, and seeds. In addition to fresh produce, it is important to include pantry staples such as whole-grain pasta, brown rice, quinoa, canned beans, and low-sodium vegetable broth, which provide a foundation for creating nourishing meals. Furthermore, incorporating herbs, spices, and condiments like turmeric, ginger, garlic, and olive oil can add flavor and depth to dishes while also offering potential health benefits.

 Proper storage of pantry items is essential to maintain their freshness and nutritional integrity, so it is advisable to store perishable items like nuts and seeds in airtight containers in a cool, dark place, while canned goods should be checked regularly for expiration dates. By stocking a pantry with a diverse array of nutrient-rich foods, individuals can ensure that they have the ingredients on hand to prepare wholesome meals that support cancer prevention and promote overall well-being.

Essential Kitchen Tools And Equipment:

Equipping a kitchen with essential tools and equipment is essential for efficiently preparing cancer-fighting meals and optimizing nutrient retention during the cooking process.

Fundamental kitchen tools include sharp knives, cutting boards, measuring cups and spoons, mixing bowls, and a variety of utensils such as spatulas, whisks, and tongs, which are necessary for chopping, slicing, measuring, mixing, and stirring ingredients. Additionally, having a well-functioning stove, oven, and microwave enables individuals to cook a wide range of foods using different methods, from sautéing and steaming to roasting and baking.

Other essential appliances include a blender or food processor for making smoothies, soups, and sauces, as well as a juicer for extracting fresh fruit and vegetable juices. Furthermore, investing in high-quality cookware such as non-stick pots and pans, baking sheets, and roasting pans can help prevent burning and sticking while minimizing the need for added fats and oils during cooking.

Kitchen equipment like a food thermometer and timer can also ensure that foods are cooked to safe temperatures and prevent overcooking or undercooking. By having the necessary tools and equipment on hand, individuals can streamline their cooking process and create delicious, nutritious meals that support cancer prevention and overall health.

Tips For Shopping For Cancer-Fighting Foods:

Navigating the grocery store with a focus on purchasing cancer-fighting foods requires careful planning and attention to detail.

One of the first tips for successful shopping is to prepare a detailed shopping list based on planned meals and recipes, which helps minimize impulse purchases and ensures that essential ingredients are not forgotten. When selecting fresh produce, it is important to choose a variety of colors and textures, as different fruits and vegetables contain unique combinations of vitamins, minerals, and antioxidants.

Opting for organic produce whenever possible can reduce exposure to pesticides and synthetic chemicals, although it is important to prioritize eating a diverse range of fruits and vegetables regardless of their organic status. In the aisles, reading food labels can help identify products that are low in added sugars, sodium, and unhealthy fats, while also looking for whole grain options and minimizing processed and packaged foods. Shopping from the perimeter of the store, where fresh produce, lean proteins, dairy, and whole grains are typically located, can help prioritize nutrient-dense foods over processed snacks and sugary beverages found in the center aisles. Additionally, buying in bulk or purchasing frozen fruits and vegetables can be cost-effective ways to incorporate more plant-based foods into the diet while reducing food waste. By following these tips and strategies, individuals can make informed choices while shopping for cancer-fighting foods and support their efforts to maintain a healthy diet that promotes overall well-being.

CHAPTER 3

BREAKFASTS TO KICKSTART YOUR DAY

Breakfast is often touted as the most important meal of the day, and for good reason. It sets the tone for your energy levels and nutritional intake throughout the day. In the context of a cancer prevention diet, breakfast becomes even more crucial as it offers an opportunity to kickstart your day with nourishing foods that support overall health and well-being. This section of the cookbook focuses on providing a variety of options that not only taste delicious but also offer a rich array of nutrients to fuel your body and mind.

Nutrient-Packed Breakfast Smoothies

Smoothies are a popular choice for breakfast as they offer a convenient way to pack in a variety of nutrients in a single serving. In the context of cancer prevention, smoothies can be particularly beneficial as they allow for the incorporation of ingredients known for their anti-inflammatory and antioxidant properties. Ingredients such as leafy greens, berries, nuts, seeds, and plant-based protein sources like tofu or pea protein can all be blended to create a nutrient-packed morning beverage. These smoothies not only provide essential vitamins and minerals but also support immune function and overall health.

Whole Grain Breakfast Bowls

Whole grains are an integral part of a balanced diet, and incorporating them into your breakfast can provide sustained energy and a feeling of fullness throughout the morning. Whole grain breakfast bowls offer a customizable option where individuals can mix and match grains, fruits, nuts, and seeds to create a satisfying meal. Examples of whole grains that can be used include oats, quinoa, barley, and brown rice, all of which are rich in fiber, vitamins, and minerals. By starting your day with a whole grain breakfast bowl, you're not only supporting your overall health but also reducing the risk of chronic diseases such as cancer.

Energizing Oatmeal Variations

Oatmeal is a classic breakfast choice that can be transformed into a variety of delicious and nutritious dishes. In the context of a cancer-prevention diet, oatmeal offers numerous health benefits, including its high fiber content, which aids in digestion and helps regulate blood sugar levels.

This section of the cookbook explores different ways to prepare oatmeal, from simple combinations with fruits and nuts to more elaborate recipes that incorporate spices and superfoods like chia seeds or flaxseeds. By incorporating oatmeal into your breakfast routine, you're not only starting your day with a hearty and satisfying meal but also providing your body with essential nutrients that support overall health and well-being.

Plant-Based Protein Breakfasts

Protein is an essential nutrient that plays a crucial role in maintaining and repairing tissues, supporting immune function, and regulating hormones. In the context of a cancer prevention diet, plant-based protein sources offer numerous benefits, including their lower saturated fat content and higher levels of fiber and antioxidants. This section of the cookbook highlights a variety of plant-based protein breakfast options, including tofu scrambles, chickpea omelettes, and lentil-based breakfast patties. These recipes not only provide a satisfying and filling meal but also help reduce the risk of chronic diseases such as cancer by promoting a diet rich in fruits, vegetables, whole grains, and legumes. By incorporating these plant-based protein breakfasts into your routine, you're not only supporting your health but also contributing to a more sustainable and environmentally friendly food system.

CHAPTER 4
NOURISHING LUNCHES

Nourishing lunches play a crucial role in maintaining a healthy diet, especially for individuals focused on cancer prevention. Within the context of the "Cancer Prevention Diet Cookbook," the concept of nourishing lunches encompasses a variety of meal options designed to provide essential nutrients while also being flavorful and satisfying. Among these options are colorful salad creations, protein-packed lunch wraps, hearty grain and vegetable bowls, and homemade soups and stews.

Each of these lunch ideas offers unique benefits in terms of nutrition, taste, and ease of preparation, contributing to a well-rounded approach to cancer prevention through dietary choices.

Colorful salad creations are a cornerstone of a nourishing lunch menu, offering a vibrant array of vegetables, fruits, and other wholesome ingredients. These salads are not only visually appealing but also rich in vitamins, minerals, and antioxidants, which are essential for maintaining overall health and reducing the risk of cancer.

By incorporating a diverse range of colorful vegetables such as leafy greens, tomatoes, bell peppers, carrots, and beets, these salads provide a spectrum of nutrients that support immune function, promote detoxification, and help combat inflammation—all of which are crucial in cancer prevention. Additionally, adding sources of plant-based protein such as legumes, nuts, seeds, or grilled tofu can enhance the nutritional profile of these salads, making them both satisfying and nourishing.

Protein-packed lunch wraps offer a convenient and portable option for individuals seeking to maintain a balanced diet while on the go. These wraps typically feature a combination of lean protein sources, such as grilled chicken, turkey, fish, or plant-based alternatives like tempeh or hummus, along with an assortment of fresh vegetables and whole grains wrapped in a whole-grain tortilla or flatbread.

By prioritizing protein-rich ingredients, these wraps provide essential amino acids necessary for cell repair and regeneration, while also offering fiber, vitamins, and minerals from the accompanying vegetables and grains. This combination of nutrients not only supports overall health and satiety but also helps to regulate blood sugar levels and promote a healthy weight, both of which are important factors in cancer prevention.

Hearty grain and vegetable bowls offer a satisfying and customizable lunch option that combines complex carbohydrates, protein, fiber, and various micronutrients in a single dish. These bowls typically feature a base of cooked whole grains such as quinoa, brown rice, or barley, topped with a colorful array of roasted or steamed vegetables, leafy greens, and protein sources such as beans, lentils, grilled tofu, or lean meats.

By incorporating a variety of plant-based foods, these bowls provide a diverse array of nutrients, including antioxidants, phytochemicals, and dietary fiber, which have been shown to have protective effects against cancer development.

Additionally, the inclusion of whole grains ensures a slow and steady release of energy, helping to maintain stable blood sugar levels and promote sustained feelings of fullness and satisfaction throughout the afternoon.

Homemade soups and stews offer a comforting and nourishing lunch option that can be prepared in advance and enjoyed throughout the week. These hearty dishes typically consist of a flavorful broth or base, combined with a variety of vegetables, legumes, whole grains, and lean proteins, simmered together to create a rich and satisfying meal.

By using wholesome, unprocessed ingredients and minimizing added salt, sugar, and unhealthy fats, homemade soups, and stews provide a nutrient-dense alternative to pre-packaged or restaurant versions, which may contain hidden additives or excessive amounts of sodium. Additionally, the slow cooking process allows for the flavors of the ingredients to meld together, resulting in a comforting and satisfying dish that can be easily customized to suit individual taste preferences and dietary needs. Overall, homemade soups and stews offer a convenient and nourishing lunch option that supports overall health and well-being, making them a valuable addition to a cancer-prevention diet.

CHAPTER 5
WHOLESOME DINNERS

The concept of wholesome dinners encompasses the idea of creating balanced, nutritious meals that support overall health and well-being, particularly in the context of cancer prevention. A wholesome dinner typically consists of a variety of nutrient-dense foods that provide essential vitamins, minerals, antioxidants, and other bioactive compounds known to promote health and reduce the risk of chronic diseases, including cancer. These meals are designed to nourish the body and support its natural defense mechanisms against cancerous growth and development.

In the context of cancer prevention, wholesome dinners often prioritize whole foods such as fruits, vegetables, whole grains, lean proteins, and healthy fats.

These foods are rich in phytochemicals, fiber, and other nutrients that have been shown to have protective effects against cancer. By incorporating a diverse range of plant-based foods into dinner recipes, individuals can ensure they are receiving a wide array of beneficial compounds that may help lower their risk of developing cancer.

Furthermore, wholesome dinners are typically prepared using cooking methods that preserve the nutritional integrity of the ingredients. Steaming, roasting, grilling, and baking are preferred over frying or deep-frying, as these methods help retain the nutrients present in the foods without adding excessive amounts of unhealthy fats or calories. Additionally, minimizing the use of processed and refined ingredients, such as white flour and sugar, is important in creating truly wholesome dinners that support optimal health and cancer prevention.

Overall, the concept of wholesome dinners emphasizes the importance of mindful eating and making informed food choices that prioritize health and well-being.

By focusing on nutrient-dense whole foods and preparing them in a way that preserves their nutritional value, individuals can harness the power of nutrition to support their fight against cancer and promote long-term health.

Flavorful One-Pot Meals:

Flavorful one-pot meals are a practical and convenient option for individuals looking to prepare nutritious dinners while minimizing time spent in the kitchen. These meals typically involve cooking all ingredients in a single pot or pan, resulting in dishes that are easy to prepare, serve, and clean up. Despite their simplicity, flavorful one-pot meals can be incredibly versatile and satisfying, offering a wide range of flavors, textures, and nutritional benefits.

In the context of cancer prevention, flavorful one-pot meals offer an opportunity to incorporate a variety of cancer-fighting ingredients into a single dish. By combining different vegetables, proteins, whole grains, herbs, and spices, individuals can create meals that are not only delicious but also packed with nutrients known to support overall health and reduce the risk of cancer. For example, incorporating cruciferous vegetables like broccoli, cauliflower, and Brussels sprouts into one-pot meals can provide a rich source of sulforaphane, a compound with potent anti-cancer properties.

Moreover, one-pot meals can be customized to suit individual dietary preferences and restrictions, making them suitable for a wide range of individuals, including those following plant-based, gluten-free, or dairy-free diets. By experimenting with different ingredient combinations and flavor profiles, individuals can discover new and exciting ways to enjoy nutritious meals that support their cancer prevention goals.

Additionally, one-pot meals are often ideal for meal prepping, allowing individuals to prepare large batches of food in advance and portion them out for easy grab-and-go meals throughout the week. This can be particularly helpful for busy individuals or those undergoing cancer treatment who may have limited time or energy to devote to cooking elaborate dinners.

flavorful one-pot meals offer a convenient and practical solution for incorporating nutritious, cancer-fighting foods into one's diet. By embracing the versatility and simplicity of these dishes, individuals can enjoy delicious meals that support their overall health and well-being while reducing their risk of cancer.

Vibrant Vegetable Stir-Fries:

Vibrant vegetable stir-fries offer a delicious and nutritious way to incorporate an abundance of colorful vegetables into one's diet while enjoying bold flavors and satisfying textures. This cooking method involves quickly sautéing bite-sized pieces of vegetables in a hot pan with a small amount of oil and seasoning them with herbs, spices, and sauces to enhance their flavor. The result is a vibrant and flavorful dish that is both visually appealing and packed with essential nutrients.

In the context of cancer prevention, vibrant vegetable stir-fries are an excellent way to increase the intake of plant-based foods, which are rich in antioxidants, vitamins, minerals, and phytochemicals that have been shown to have protective effects against cancer. By including a variety of colorful vegetables such as bell peppers, broccoli, carrots, spinach, and mushrooms, individuals can ensure they are receiving a wide range of beneficial nutrients that support overall health and well-being.

Moreover, vegetable stir-fries can be easily customized to suit individual tastes and dietary preferences. For example, individuals can choose to add lean proteins such as chicken, tofu, or shrimp to their stir-fries for added protein and satiety, or they can keep the dish entirely plant-based by using ingredients like tofu or tempeh as the main protein source. Additionally, individuals can adjust the seasoning and sauce ingredients to suit their flavor preferences and dietary restrictions, making vegetable stir-fries a versatile and adaptable option for any meal.

Furthermore, vegetable stir-fries are quick and easy to prepare, making them an ideal choice for busy weeknights or hectic schedules. With just a few simple ingredients and minimal cooking time, individuals can whip up a delicious and nutritious meal that satisfies hunger and provides essential nutrients to support their overall health and well-being.

vibrant vegetable stir-fries offer a convenient and delicious way to incorporate a variety of colorful vegetables into one's diet while enjoying bold flavors and satisfying textures. By embracing this cooking method and experimenting with different ingredient combinations, individuals can enjoy nutritious meals that support their cancer prevention goals and promote overall health and well-being.

Grilled and baked fish dishes offer a delicious and nutritious way to incorporate lean protein and essential omega-3 fatty acids into one's diet while enjoying the distinct flavors and textures of seafood. These cooking methods involve cooking fish fillets or whole fish on a grill or in the oven with minimal added fat, resulting in dishes that are light, flavorful, and packed with essential nutrients.

In the context of cancer prevention, grilled and baked fish dishes are particularly beneficial due to the high concentration of omega-3 fatty acids found in fatty fish such as salmon, mackerel, and sardines.

Omega-3 fatty acids have been shown to have anti-inflammatory properties and may help reduce the risk of certain types of cancer, including breast, prostate, and colorectal cancer. Additionally, fish is a rich source of high-quality protein and essential vitamins and minerals, making it an excellent choice for supporting overall health and well-being.

Moreover, grilled and baked fish dishes are incredibly versatile and can be prepared using a variety of seasonings, marinades, and sauces to suit individual tastes and preferences. For example, individuals can marinate fish fillets in a mixture of citrus juice, herbs, and spices before grilling or baking them for added flavor and tenderness.

 Similarly, a simple sprinkle of salt, pepper, and lemon juice can enhance the natural flavors of the fish without overpowering its delicate taste.

Additionally, grilled and baked fish dishes are quick and easy to prepare, making them an ideal option for busy weeknights or hectic schedules. With just a few simple ingredients and minimal cooking time, individuals can create a delicious and nutritious meal that is sure to satisfy hunger and provide essential nutrients to support their overall health and well-being.

CHAPTER 6

Snacks and appetizers play a significant role in our daily dietary intake, contributing to our overall nutritional intake and satiety levels. In the context of a cancer-prevention diet, these snacks and appetizers can serve as crucial components in promoting health and well-being. This section focuses on various snack and appetizer options tailored to support cancer prevention through the incorporation of nutrient-dense ingredients and mindful culinary choices.

Fresh Fruit and Veggie Snack Ideas: Incorporating fresh fruits and vegetables into snack choices offers numerous health benefits, particularly in the context of cancer prevention. Fruits and vegetables are rich in vitamins, minerals, antioxidants, and dietary fiber, all of which play vital roles in maintaining cellular health and supporting the body's natural defense mechanisms against cancer development. Examples of fresh fruit and veggie snack ideas include sliced apples with almond butter, carrot sticks with hummus, or a colorful fruit salad. These snacks not only provide essential nutrients but also offer a refreshing and satisfying option for those seeking to incorporate more plant-based foods into their diet.

Nutrient-Dense Trail Mixes: Trail mixes are versatile snacks that can be customized to include a variety of nutrient-dense ingredients such as nuts, seeds, dried fruits, and whole grains. Nuts and seeds are excellent sources of healthy fats, protein, and essential micronutrients like vitamin E and magnesium, which have been linked to reduced cancer risk.

Additionally, dried fruits add natural sweetness and fiber to the mix, while whole grains contribute complex carbohydrates for sustained energy. By choosing ingredients rich in antioxidants and anti-inflammatory compounds, such as walnuts and dark chocolate, trail mixes can provide a convenient and nourishing snack option that supports cancer prevention efforts.

Homemade Hummus and Dips: Hummus and other homemade dips offer a flavorful and nutritious alternative to store-bought options that may contain additives and preservatives. Chickpeas, the primary ingredient in hummus, are a good source of protein, fiber, and folate, which are important for maintaining cellular health and supporting immune function. By making hummus at home, individuals can control the ingredients and customize flavors to suit their preferences. Incorporating ingredients like garlic, lemon juice, and tahini not only enhances the taste but also adds additional health-promoting properties, such as antimicrobial and anti-inflammatory effects. Pairing homemade hummus with fresh vegetables or whole-grain crackers creates a balanced snack option that promotes satiety and provides essential nutrients for cancer prevention.

Guilt-Free Sweet Treats: While it's important to limit the consumption of refined sugars and processed sweets in a cancer-prevention diet, there are still plenty of guilt-free sweet treat options available. By using natural sweeteners like honey, maple syrup, or dates, individuals can satisfy their sweet cravings while also benefiting from the nutritional value of these alternatives. For example, homemade energy balls made with oats, nuts, dried fruits, and a touch of natural sweetener provide a satisfying snack that delivers a mix of carbohydrates, protein, and healthy fats. Similarly, frozen banana slices dipped in dark chocolate offer a decadent yet nutritious treat rich in antioxidants and potassium. By opting for homemade sweet treats made with wholesome ingredients, individuals can indulge in moderation without compromising their cancer prevention efforts.

CHAPTER 7
SIDES AND ACCOMPANIMENTS

Colorful Vegetable Side Dishes:

In the context of the "Cancer Prevention Diet Cookbook," the inclusion of colorful vegetable side dishes serves multiple purposes, all aligned with the overarching goal of cancer prevention and management through nutrition. Vegetables, particularly those vibrant in color, are rich in essential vitamins, minerals, antioxidants, and phytochemicals, which play crucial roles in bolstering the body's defense mechanisms against cancerous growth. These side dishes not only add visual appeal to meals but also contribute significantly to the nutritional profile, offering a diverse array of nutrients that support overall health and well-being.

The emphasis on color in vegetable selection is not merely aesthetic; rather, it reflects the diversity of nutrients present in different plant-based foods. For instance, red and orange vegetables like tomatoes, carrots, and bell peppers are abundant in carotenoids such as beta-carotene and lycopene, known for their antioxidant properties. These compounds help neutralize harmful free radicals in the body, thereby reducing oxidative stress and the risk of cellular damage that could lead to cancer development. Similarly, green leafy vegetables like spinach, kale, and broccoli boast high levels of vitamins C and K, folate, and various phytonutrients, all of which contribute to cellular repair and immune function.

Furthermore, incorporating a variety of colorful vegetables into side dishes ensures a broad spectrum of micronutrients, each with its unique health-promoting benefits. For example, cruciferous vegetables like cauliflower, Brussels sprouts, and cabbage contain sulfur-containing compounds such as glycosylates, which have been studied for their potential anticancer effects, including detoxification of carcinogens and inhibition of tumor growth.

By including such diverse options in vegetable side dishes, individuals can optimize their nutrient intake and enhance their body's resilience against cancer and other chronic diseases.

Moreover, these colorful vegetable side dishes offer practical and flavorful alternatives to less nutritious accompaniments, such as refined grains or high-fat, high-calorie options.

By focusing on whole, minimally processed plant foods, individuals can maintain a diet that is rich in fiber, vitamins, and minerals while minimizing the intake of added sugars, unhealthy fats, and preservatives—factors that have been linked to an increased risk of cancer and other adverse health outcomes.

Thus, these side dishes not only enhance the nutritional quality of meals but also promote sustainable dietary habits that support long-term health and disease prevention.

the inclusion of colorful vegetable side dishes in the "Cancer Prevention Diet Cookbook" underscores the critical role of plant-based nutrition in mitigating cancer risk and promoting overall well-being.

By harnessing the diverse array of nutrients and phytochemicals found in different vegetables, individuals can support their body's natural defense mechanisms and create meals that are both nourishing and delicious.

Moreover, these side dishes offer practical alternatives to less healthy accompaniments, reinforcing the importance of whole, minimally processed foods in cancer prevention and management.

CHAPTER 8
DESSERTS WITH BENEFITS

In the context of the "Cancer Prevention Diet Cookbook," the concept of "Desserts with Benefits" embodies a paradigm shift in the perception of desserts.

Traditionally viewed as indulgent, calorie-laden treats with little nutritional value, desserts are redefined in this cookbook as vehicles for delivering health-promoting ingredients. Desserts with Benefits prioritize the incorporation of nutrient-dense ingredients such as fruits, whole grains, nuts, and antioxidants, thereby transforming desserts into nourishing components of a balanced diet.

This approach not only satisfies the sweet cravings but also contributes to overall health and well-being by providing essential vitamins, minerals, fiber, and phytochemicals. By reimagining desserts as functional foods, this concept aligns with the broader ethos of the cookbook, which emphasizes the proactive role of nutrition in cancer prevention and management.

Fruit-Focused Dessert Recipes:

Fruit-focused dessert recipes epitomize the fusion of taste and health in the "Cancer Prevention Diet Cookbook." Fruits are renowned for their abundance of vitamins, minerals, fiber, and antioxidants, making them integral components of a cancer-preventive diet. In this section, the cookbook showcases a diverse array of dessert recipes that highlight the natural sweetness and versatility of fruits.

From vibrant berry compotes to refreshing citrus sorbets and decadent grilled peaches, these recipes celebrate the inherent flavors and nutritional benefits of fruits.

Moreover, by incorporating fruits into desserts, individuals can satisfy their sweet cravings while simultaneously reaping the health-enhancing properties of these nutrient-rich ingredients. By promoting fruit-focused dessert recipes, the cookbook encourages individuals to embrace a dietary pattern that prioritizes whole, plant-based foods as a cornerstone of cancer prevention and overall well-being.

Whole Grain And Nut-Based Desserts:

Whole grain and nut-based desserts represent a departure from traditional dessert formulations characterized by refined flour and sugars. Instead, these desserts harness the nutritional power of whole grains and nuts to deliver sustained energy, satiety, and essential nutrients.

Whole grains such as oats, quinoa, and brown rice provide fiber, vitamins, minerals, and antioxidants, while nuts like almonds, walnuts, and pistachios offer healthy fats, protein, and micronutrients.

By incorporating these wholesome ingredients into dessert recipes, the cookbook not only enhances the nutritional profile but also promotes dietary patterns associated with reduced cancer risk. Furthermore, whole grain and nut-based desserts offer a satisfying texture and depth of flavor, making them equally—if not more—appealing than their conventional counterparts. As such, this concept underscores the notion that desserts can be both delicious and nutritious, reinforcing the cookbook's overarching message of leveraging food as a tool for cancer prevention and support.

The notion of guilt-free indulgences encapsulates the philosophy of balance and moderation espoused by the "Cancer Prevention Diet Cookbook." Contrary to the perception that indulgent desserts must be accompanied by feelings of guilt or remorse, this concept emphasizes the importance of enjoying treats mindfully and responsibly. Guilt-free indulgences in the context of the cookbook refer to desserts that offer satisfaction and pleasure without compromising health goals or exacerbating cancer risk factors. By utilizing wholesome ingredients and mindful portion control, individuals can indulge in desserts guilt-free, knowing that they are nourishing their bodies and supporting overall well-being. Moreover, the cookbook provides guidance on incorporating indulgences into a balanced diet, emphasizing the importance of variety, moderation, and self-awareness. Through this approach, guilt-free indulgences empower individuals to cultivate a positive relationship with food, free from the constraints of guilt or deprivation, thereby promoting long-term dietary adherence and sustainable lifestyle habits.

Sweet Treats With Antioxidant Power:

Sweet treats with antioxidant power exemplify the intersection of flavor and functionality in the "Cancer Prevention Diet Cookbook." Antioxidants, compounds found in foods such as fruits, vegetables, nuts, and spices, play a crucial role in neutralizing harmful free radicals and reducing oxidative stress, thereby mitigating the risk of cancer development and progression. By incorporating ingredients rich in antioxidants—such as dark chocolate, berries, green tea, and turmeric—into dessert recipes, the cookbook elevates the health-promoting potential of sweet treats. These antioxidant-rich desserts not only satisfy the palate but also serve as potent allies in the fight against cancer, offering a delicious way to fortify the body's defense mechanisms. Moreover, the inclusion of antioxidants adds depth of flavor, complexity, and visual appeal to desserts, enhancing their sensory allure and culinary experience. As such, sweet treats with antioxidant power exemplify the synergy between taste and health, reinforcing the cookbook's overarching mission of harnessing the power of nutrition in the prevention and management of cancer.

CHAPTER 9
BEVERAGES FOR HEALTH

Beverages for Health play a significant role in promoting overall well-being and supporting specific health objectives, such as cancer prevention and management. Within the context of the "Cancer Prevention Diet Cookbook," these beverages are carefully curated to provide nourishment and support to individuals seeking to harness the power of nutrition in their fight against cancer. The inclusion of Hydrating Infusions and Teas reflects a commitment to hydration, a fundamental aspect of health maintenance. These beverages are often infused with herbs, fruits, or vegetables, imparting not only hydration but also valuable nutrients and antioxidants. Herbal teas, such as green tea or chamomile, are known for their antioxidant properties, which can help reduce inflammation and oxidative stress, factors associated with cancer development and progression. Furthermore, infusions utilizing ingredients like cucumber, mint, or citrus fruits offer refreshing flavors while contributing essential vitamins and minerals to the diet.

Nutrient-rich smoothies and Juices are another cornerstone of the cancer prevention diet, offering a convenient and delicious way to incorporate a variety of nutrients into one's daily routine. Smoothies, typically made with a base of fruits and vegetables blended with liquids like water, coconut water, or plant-based milk, provide a concentrated source of vitamins, minerals, fiber, and phytonutrients. These beverages can be tailored to individual preferences and nutritional needs, with ingredients chosen for their specific health-promoting properties.

For instance, berries are rich in antioxidants like anthocyanins, while leafy greens offer ample amounts of folate and vitamin K. Additionally, the inclusion of ingredients like flaxseeds or chia seeds can provide omega-3 fatty acids, which have been linked to reduced inflammation and improved overall health outcomes.

Healing Herbal Tonics represents a traditional approach to health and wellness, harnessing the therapeutic properties of herbs and botanicals to support the body's natural healing processes. These tonics often feature ingredients with adaptogenic or immune-modulating effects, such as echinacea, astragalus, or medicinal mushrooms like reishi or shiitake.

By incorporating these ingredients into beverages, individuals can benefit from their potential anti-cancer properties, including enhanced immune function and reduced inflammation. Herbal tonics may also include ingredients known for their detoxifying or liver-supportive properties, such as dandelion root or milk thistle, which can aid in the body's natural detoxification processes and support overall health.

Alcohol-free mocktails offer a healthy and enjoyable alternative to traditional cocktails, providing all the flavor and sophistication without the negative health effects associated with alcohol consumption.

In the context of cancer prevention, avoiding or reducing alcohol intake is often recommended due to its potential carcinogenic effects, particularly concerning breast, liver, and colorectal cancers. Mocktails provide a satisfying alternative for individuals looking to socialize or celebrate without compromising their health goals. These beverages can be crafted using a variety of ingredients, including fresh fruits, herbs, sparkling water, and non-alcoholic spirits or bitters, allowing for endless creativity and customization. By incorporating vibrant flavors and nutritious ingredients, alcohol-free mocktails contribute to a well-rounded cancer prevention diet, supporting overall health and vitality.

CHAPTER 10
MEAL PLANNING AND TIPS FOR LONG-TERM SUCCESS

Meal planning is a cornerstone of any successful dietary regimen, particularly in the context of cancer prevention.

A thoughtful approach to meal planning can not only ensure that individuals consume a balanced diet but also facilitate adherence to dietary guidelines over the long term.

It involves the strategic selection of ingredients and recipes to meet nutritional goals while accommodating individual preferences and dietary restrictions.

A key aspect of meal planning for cancer prevention is the emphasis on whole, nutrient-dense foods such as fruits, vegetables, whole grains, lean proteins, and healthy fats while minimizing processed foods, sugar, and saturated fats.

 By incorporating a variety of colorful fruits and vegetables, individuals can benefit from a diverse array of vitamins, minerals, antioxidants, and phytochemicals, which have been shown to have protective effects against cancer.

Strategies For Meal Prep And Batch Cooking:

Meal prep and batch cooking are invaluable strategies for busy individuals seeking to maintain a healthy diet while minimizing time spent in the kitchen. By dedicating a few hours each week to preparing meals in advance, individuals can streamline their cooking process, reduce food waste, and ensure access to nutritious meals throughout the week. This approach involves planning and preparing larger quantities of food at once, which can then be portioned out and stored for later consumption. For cancer prevention, batch cooking allows individuals to focus on incorporating a variety of cancer-fighting ingredients into their meals, such as cruciferous vegetables, leafy greens, legumes, and lean proteins. Additionally, by prepping healthy snacks and convenience foods, individuals can resist the temptation of reaching for less nutritious options when hunger strikes.

Creating Balanced Cancer Prevention Meal Plans:

Creating balanced meal plans tailored to cancer prevention requires careful consideration of nutritional needs, dietary preferences, and lifestyle factors.

A balanced diet for cancer prevention should include a variety of foods from all food groups, with an emphasis on plant-based foods such as fruits, vegetables, whole grains, nuts, seeds, and legumes.

These foods are rich in vitamins, minerals, fiber, and antioxidants, which play key roles in reducing inflammation, supporting immune function, and protecting against cellular damage that can lead to cancer. Additionally, incorporating lean sources of protein, such as poultry, fish, tofu, and legumes, can help maintain muscle mass and support overall health. Whole foods should be prioritized over processed and refined options, as they tend to be higher in nutrients and lower in added sugars, salt, and unhealthy fats.

Tips For Dining Out And Social Occasions:

Dining out and social occasions can present challenges for individuals following a cancer-prevention diet, as they often involve exposure to less healthy food options and peer pressure to indulge in indulgent foods and drinks. However, with careful planning and mindful decision-making, it is possible to navigate these situations while staying true to dietary goals.

One strategy is to research restaurant menus in advance and choose establishments that offer healthy options, such as salads, grilled proteins, and vegetable-based dishes.

Additionally, individuals can communicate their dietary preferences and restrictions to restaurant staff to ensure that meals are prepared to their specifications. When attending social gatherings, bringing a nutritious dish to share can ensure that there are healthy options available, while also inspiring others to make healthier choices. It's also important to practice mindful eating and enjoy indulgent foods in moderation, rather than feeling deprived or guilty.

Staying Motivated On Your Cancer Prevention Journey:

Maintaining motivation on the cancer prevention journey requires a combination of self-awareness, goal-setting, social support, and positive reinforcement. Individuals need to identify their reasons for prioritizing cancer prevention, whether it's to improve overall health, reduce cancer risk factors, or support loved ones who have been affected by the disease.

Setting realistic, achievable goals and tracking progress can provide a sense of accomplishment and motivation to continue making healthy choices. Surrounding oneself with supportive friends, family members, or online communities can also provide encouragement, accountability, and inspiration.

Celebrating milestones, no matter how small, and rewarding oneself for progress can help reinforce positive behaviors and maintain momentum on the journey toward cancer prevention. Additionally, practicing self-care, stress management, and mindfulness techniques can help individuals cope with challenges and setbacks along the way, allowing them to stay focused on their long-term health goals. Ultimately, staying motivated on the cancer prevention journey requires commitment, resilience, and a willingness to prioritize health and well-being.

CONCLUSION

Cancer Prevention Diet Cookbook," the central focus lies on the pivotal role of nutrition in combating cancer.

This comprehensive guide offers a plethora of nourishing recipes and expert guidance, aimed at empowering individuals to harness the power of nutrition in their fight against cancer. The title itself, "Cancer Prevention Diet Cookbook," underscores the proactive approach to cancer prevention through dietary choices. It suggests that diet plays a crucial role not only in preventing cancer but also in supporting those undergoing treatment. The subtitle, "Nourishing Recipes and Expert Guidance for Harnessing the Power of Nutrition in Your Fight Against Cancer," further elaborates on the contents of the book, indicating that it offers both practical recipes and authoritative advice from experts in the field of oncology and nutrition.

The concept of cancer prevention through diet is a multifaceted one, encompassing various dietary components and their interactions with the body's mechanisms. This includes understanding the role of antioxidants, phytochemicals, vitamins, and minerals in neutralizing free radicals and reducing inflammation, which are processes implicated in cancer development.

The cookbook delves into the science behind these dietary elements, providing readers with a deeper understanding of how specific nutrients can help prevent cancer or support treatment outcomes.

Moreover, the cookbook emphasizes the importance of adopting a balanced and diverse diet rich in fruits, vegetables, whole grains, lean proteins, and healthy fats.

It encourages readers to explore a wide array of ingredients and culinary techniques to create flavorful and nutritious meals that promote overall health and well-being.

By incorporating a variety of foods into their diet, individuals can ensure they are obtaining essential nutrients that support immune function, promote detoxification, and maintain optimal cellular health – all of which are crucial in cancer prevention and management.

Additionally, the cookbook addresses the role of lifestyle factors such as physical activity, stress management, and adequate sleep in cancer prevention. It highlights the interconnectedness of diet, lifestyle, and cancer risk, underscoring the importance of adopting a holistic approach to health. Through practical tips and strategies, readers are encouraged to make sustainable changes to their lifestyle that support overall health and reduce cancer risk.

Furthermore, the cookbook provides practical tools and resources to help readers implement dietary and lifestyle changes effectively. This may include meal planning guides, grocery shopping lists, cooking tips, and meal prep strategies to make healthy eating more accessible and convenient. By empowering readers with the knowledge and skills to navigate dietary choices confidently, the cookbook aims to promote long-term adherence to a cancer-preventive diet and lifestyle.

In conclusion, the "Cancer Prevention Diet Cookbook" serves as a comprehensive resource for individuals looking to harness the power of nutrition in their fight against cancer. By offering nourishing recipes, expert guidance, and practical tools, the cookbook empowers readers to make informed dietary and lifestyle choices that support cancer prevention and improve overall well-being.

Through a holistic approach that addresses the interplay between diet, lifestyle, and cancer risk, this cookbook provides readers with the knowledge and resources they need to take control of their health and reduce their risk of cancer.

www.ingramcontent.com/pod-product-compliance
Lightning Source LLC
Chambersburg PA
CBHW060755260726
48660CB00002B/629